Proxy Information For You And Your Healthcare Agent

Pierre Mouchette

Life Knowledge Media USA
An Enviro | Life Knowledge Publication
a subsidiary of Real Property Experts LLC

ISBN 979 - 8814539342 (Paperback Book)

Independently Published

First Edition: May 2022
Life Knowledge Media USA
An Enviro | Life Knowledge Publication
Web Address: https://www.enviro-life-media.com
Contact: publications@synchronicity-investor.com

Note: This publication comes in various formats, such as Paperbacks and Electronic Books (e-books). Some material in the paperback version of this book may not be included in e-books, and vice versa.

At Life Knowledge Media USA, we pride ourselves on every publication's quality, research, and transparency. All content is carefully researched.

DISCLAIMER

This Life Knowledge Media USA publication provides information about the subject matter covered. The author and publisher of this content are not acting as licensed professionals to present the covered material. The information and statements made are for educational purposes and are not intended to replace a one-on-one relationship with a qualified attorney, accountant, tax professional, or other licensed professionals. You are solely responsible for the use of any content. You hold Real Property Experts LLC, its subsidiaries, and members harmless in any event or claim, demand, or damage, including reasonable attorneys' fees, asserted by any third party, or arising out of your use of, or conduct on, publications and products.

Life Knowledge Media USA writers provide applicable content and break down complex topics so they are easier to understand. Information given may not apply to your specific situation, and products or services recommended may not be a good fit for your application. While Life Knowledge Media USA strives to provide accurate, up-to-date content, we cannot guarantee the accuracy and completeness of the information supplied. By using this content, you understand that all material is an expression of opinion and not professional advice.

PREFACE

A **Healthcare Proxy (HCP)** is a legal document (instrument) in which the **Grantor** or **Principal** engages a **Healthcare Agent** to make health care decisions on their behalf when they are incapable of making and executing their own health care decisions.

Once the healthcare proxy is effective, the Agent continues making health care decisions as long as the **Principal** is legally incompetent to decide. The document also discloses the authority given by the **Grantor** or **Principal** to the Healthcare Agent and states the limitations of this authority.

Understanding and implementing the guidelines herein is not an overnight task. Please read the contents of this publication and start planning your HCP in conjunction with your legal advisor. The information provided is for educational purposes. The objective of this book is not to provide legal advice or exhaustive coverage for all possible situations but to provide a foundation to develop further understanding.

For comments on this publication, please write to us at publications@rpe4u.com.

Contents

In life, you never know what may happen in the future. It can take a second for your life to change dramatically, including when it comes to your health and welfare. This can be hard to imagine when you are in good health, and often we do not want to imagine a time when that will not be the case.

However, since circumstances can change instantly, it is a wise decision to plan and prepare for the uncertainties in life. Choosing a Healthcare Agent is one way to document your health care directives in advance legally.

Pierre Mouchette, author

Chapter 1
YOUR HEALTHCARE PROXY

What Is A Healthcare Proxy?

A Healthcare Proxy (HCP) is a legal document that gives the 'Agent' statutory authority to make medical decisions for the Grantor or Principal. It differs from the power of attorney because it deals specifically with health care. It only comes into effect when the **Principal** can no longer make medical decisions or cannot speak or communicate their wishes. The person appointed is called a **Healthcare Agent.**

Typically, couples will name each other **Primary Healthcare Agents** and name another person as a backup. Without a healthcare proxy in place, a loved one may have to go to court to have a guardian named to direct health care treatment.

If not the spouse, the Principal may choose a family member, close friend, or attorney. The Principal may not select a doctor or a medical staff member. Additionally, the Principal may choose an **Alternate Healthcare Agent** if the **Primary Healthcare Agent** cannot decide or perform for the Principal.

If you want someone to be your Healthcare Agent, you must appoint them by filling out a Healthcare Proxy (HCP). If you do not, they will not have the legal right to make decisions for you, and a medical team will not listen to their choices.

Examples of some situations where the Healthcare Agent may need to make medical decisions include:

- Alzheimer's disease or advanced dementia

- Brain death

- Coma

- Communicating with family members about the principal's condition and treatment plan

- Deciding on medical care, medical tests, medications, and surgery

- Permitting or refusing medication, procedure, and pain management

- Pre-existing mental conditions

- Requesting or declining life-support treatments

- Requesting opinions or alternative medical care/treatment options

- Reviewing the Principal's medical history/chart

- Selecting which hospital, medical facility, nursing home, or hospice is best

- Significant memory loss

- Understanding and asking questions about the Principal's condition, and available treatment options

Common Elements of a Proxy Form

Primary Healthcare Agent - name, home address, and mobile telephone number
Function - the Primary Healthcare Agent is to make all health care decisions for the Principal, except to the extent stated otherwise. The proxy shall take effect only when and if the Principal becomes unable to make their own healthcare decisions.

Alternate Healthcare Agent - name, home address, and mobile telephone number
Function - if the **Primary Healthcare Agent** the Principal appoints is unable, unwilling, or unavailable to act as the Primary Healthcare Agent, the Principal assigns (name) an **Alternate Healthcare Agent** to make all health care decisions, except to the extent stated.

Unless the Principal revokes or states an expiration date or circumstances under which the agency will expire, this HCP shall remain indefinitely. (*Optional: If you want the proxy to expire, state the date or conditions*). This HCP shall expire (specify date or conditions):

Optional: I direct my Healthcare Agent to make health care decisions according to my wishes and limitations, as they know or as stated below. (*If you wish to limit the Agent's authority to make health care decisions or give specific instructions, express your wishes or limitations*). I direct my Healthcare Agent to make health care decisions under the following restrictions and instructions.

To make health care decisions about artificial nutrition and hydration, your Agent must know your wishes. Tell your Agent what your wishes are and include them in the Healthcare Proxy.

Optional: Organ and Tissue Bestowment

To make an anatomical gift, effective upon death, you must declare if it is for:

- Any needed organs and tissues, or

- The following organs and tissues:

____

How To Change Your Healthcare Proxy

Sometimes your thoughts change about your health care wishes or your relationship with your Healthcare Agent changes, and you want to choose another person with whom you are more comfortable. If you decide to change, follow these steps:

1) If your spouse was your Healthcare Agent and you divorced, your Healthcare Proxy (HCP) is immediately canceled.

2) Notify (either orally or in writing) your Healthcare Agent, the health care team, and family members of this change.

3) Destroy any copies of the previous Healthcare Proxy.

4) Write a new Healthcare Proxy (HCP) with the name of the new Healthcare Agent. Sign and date the new Healthcare Proxy and have two witnesses sign and date the document.

Chapter 2
YOUR HEALTHCARE AGENT

A Healthcare Agent is sometimes referred to as:

- Healthcare Surrogate

- Healthcare Representative

- Healthcare Attorney-in-Fact

What Is the Responsibility of a Healthcare Agent?

The sole role and responsibility of the Healthcare Agent will be to make all health care-related decisions should the Principal (being represented) become unable to do so for themselves. In other words, it will be the Healthcare Agent's responsibility to make essential health care decisions, including end-of-life decisions, on the Principals behalf and in the manner that they prefer. If there will be decisions to make that were previously undiscussed, the Healthcare Agent will have the task of making these decisions using their discernment. They will become their **'Principals Healthcare Advocate,'** acting as their stand-in and voice in all medical-related choices when necessary.

Because the chosen representative will be making all medical decisions as your named Healthcare Agent, you must discuss all preferences in advance so they can act as you would want them to.

What Rights Does The Healthcare Agent Have?

The rights of the Healthcare Agent can vary depending on the state. However, the most common rights include:

- Access to medical records

- Authority to approve or disapprove diagnostic tests, surgical procedures, and medication programs

- Authority to approve, withhold or withdraw artificial nutrition and hydration and all other forms of health care, including cardiopulmonary resuscitation (CPR)

- Right to choose or discharge health care providers and institutions

- The authority to sign up for organ donation, authorize an autopsy, and direct disposition of remains

- The right to consent or refuse approval to any care, treatment, service, or procedure that would impact a physical or mental condition

Why Should You Appoint A Healthcare Agent?

One of the primary benefits of appointing a Healthcare Agent is to give the Principal and their family peace of mind concerning medical care. Healthcare Agents remove or minimize much of the struggle and confusion during stressful times.

For example, family members can disagree on the type of medical treatment their loved one should receive. It can lead to arguments and issues that may escalate and require legal intervention. Doctors will consult with one individual (Healthcare Agent) to make decisions instead of waiting on a group of individuals to agree.

Another benefit of appointing a Healthcare Agent is that it can provide the ability to manage health care choices. For instance, when an Advance Directive is created, the Healthcare Agent must follow the Principal's wishes defined in the document. If a healthcare directive has not been completed, the Healthcare Agent will make decisions based upon the wishes of the Principal they are representing. Those wishes should be discussed with the appointed Healthcare Agent when the Principal is mentally and physically capable. It allows the Principal to still have a say in their medical care even when they are not competent at the time. It also eliminates much of the speculation and guesswork involved in medical care decisions.

How To Choose The Right Person

Selecting a Healthcare Agent can be difficult because it is a great responsibility to give to someone. Choosing the best person to take on the responsibility can be challenging.

The following are some items to consider when choosing a Healthcare Agent:

- **Age** - it is essential to appoint someone 18 years or older so that they can legally make decisions for their Principal.

- **Closeness** - it is best to choose a Healthcare Agent who is a close friend or family member you trust. This makes it easy to have difficult conversations and helps them understand and honor any conveyed wishes. Therefore, many individuals choose a family member such as their spouse or children. However, this is not required. Friends or legal representatives can be assigned as a Healthcare Agent.

- **Reliability** - choose someone committed to their position as your Healthcare Agent. The Agent must be reachable to make decisions. For instance, in an accident, the Healthcare Agent must be contacted as soon as possible as decisions can be time-sensitive.

- **Willingness to advocate** - a Healthcare Agent should be willing to follow any expressed wishes, even to go against the wishes of a family member. Still, if a Principal has conveyed that they do not want specific services, the Healthcare Agent should be willing to honor and advocate that decision.

- **Good communicator** - a Healthcare Agent communicates with family members with sensitivity and efficiency.

- **Willingness to make difficult decisions** - in some cases, Healthcare Agents may be required to make life or death decisions. Therefore, they must be prepared to do what is best for a person even when under emotional distress.

The Healthcare Agent

Deciding on whom you want to choose as your Healthcare Agent is not easy. This trusted person will have the authority and final say over your medical decision-making if you can no longer be responsible for them. You want to make sure you spend time thinking over whom you want to choose and ask yourself the following questions:

- **Do I Trust Them With My Life?**
  You will need to ask yourself the first and foremost question: **Who do you trust most to make life-critical decisions?** Are you confident they will make decisions in your best interests? Your life will be in the hands of your appointed Healthcare Agent.

- **Will They Be Comfortable With The Responsibility?**
  You put someone in a difficult position when deciding to make them your Healthcare Agent, especially regarding end-of-life decisions, because:
  o   You might have determined that you do not want any extraordinary measures to prolong your life.

  o   You might decide that life support should be withdrawn if you are clinically diagnosed with brain death or permanent incapacity.

  Your Healthcare Agent is responsible for ensuring that your health directives are met, even if they disagree with the choices you want them to make on your behalf. It is vital to choose someone who will be comfortable and capable of conducting your directives.

- **What Conversations Should You Have With The Prospective Healthcare Agent?**
  Once someone has agreed to accept the role as your Healthcare Agent, it will be wise for you and your Healthcare Agent to sit down and go over all healthcare decisions that your Healthcare Agent may have to make and how you would like them to be managed. A few questions you will want to cover include, but are not limited to:
  o   Do you want extraordinary measures?

  o   If you should require a skilled-nursing care facility, do you have any specific facilities in mind?

  o   Which medications are you allergic to?

  o   Who in your family or what friends do you want to access your medical records?

- Apart from the above, it is recommended that you discuss the following:
  o   Allergies, food/medicine, etc.

  o   Any religious or spiritual wishes

  o   Chronic Conditions, any ongoing medical conditions

  o   Current Medications, when/why

  o   Deciding on long-term medical care plans

  o   Decisions on surgeries and medical tests

- End of life wishes

- If you need to relocate to an assisted living, nursing home, or hospice facility

- Life-support therapies that you would or would not want to receive

- Medical medications that you would prefer not to receive, and why

- Previous surgeries, when/why

- Staying in touch with your medical team and answering their questions

- Staying up to date with your medical information

- What your feelings are concerning mechanical breathing (respirator), cardiopulmonary resuscitation (CPR), artificial nutrition and hydration, hospital intensive care, pain management, chemo or radiation therapy, and surgery

- When to decline life-support

- Which medications you can take

- Would you rather be at home or in a hospital or hospice environment

- Would you want antibiotics if you developed a life-threatening infection

Be sure to cover all healthcare directives and carefully account for all decisions.

Frequently Asked Questions

Why Choose a Healthcare Agent

If you become incapable, even temporarily, of making health care decisions, someone else must decide for you. Health care providers frequently look to family members for guidance. Family members may express what they believe your wishes are related to a particular treatment. Appointing a **Healthcare Agent** lets you control your medical treatment by:

- Choosing one person to avoid conflict and confusion among family members

- Allowing your **Healthcare Agent** to make health care decisions on your behalf as you would want them to decide

You may also appoint an **Alternate Healthcare Agent** to take over if your first choice cannot make decisions for you.

Who Could Be a Healthcare Agent

Anyone 18 years of age or older can be a Healthcare Agent. The individuals you appoint as your Healthcare Agent or your Alternate Healthcare Agent cannot sign as a witness on your Healthcare Proxy (HCP).

Whom Can I Appoint as My Healthcare Agent?

You can appoint any competent adult, 18 years of age or older, as your Healthcare Agent by having them sign the **Healthcare Proxy (HCL) form.** An attorney (although recommended) is not required, nor is a notary, Just two adult witnesses.

Note: your Healthcare Agent cannot sign as a witness.

When Does My Healthcare Agent Start Making Healthcare Decisions?

Your Healthcare Agent begins to make healthcare decisions after your doctor declares that you cannot make your own healthcare decisions. When you can make healthcare decisions again, you will be able to do so again.

What Decisions Can My Healthcare Agent Make?

Unless you limit their authority, your Healthcare Agent will be able to make any health care decision you could have made if you were able to decide for yourself. Your Healthcare Agent can agree that you should receive treatment, choose among different treatments, and decide that treatments should not be provided according to your wishes and interests. However, your Healthcare Agent can only decide on artificial nutrition and hydration (nourishment and water provided by feeding tube or intravenous line) if they know your wishes from what you have written.

Why Appoint A Healthcare Agent If I Am Young And Healthy?

If you are not elderly or terminally ill, appointing a Healthcare Agent is good. A Healthcare Agent will act on your behalf if you should become temporarily unable to make your own health care decisions. For example, you are going under general anesthesia or become comatose due to an accident. When you can make your own healthcare decisions, your Healthcare Agent will no longer be authorized to act.

How Does My Healthcare Agent Make Decisions?

Your Healthcare Agent must follow your wishes and your moral and religious beliefs. You may write specific instructions on your Healthcare Proxy (HCP) form.

How Does My Healthcare Agent Know My Wishes?

Having an open and frank discussion regarding your wishes will place your Healthcare Agent in a better position to serve your interests. If your Healthcare Agent does not know your needs or beliefs, your Healthcare Agent is legally obligated to act in what they believe to be your best interest. Because this is a crucial responsibility for the person you appoint as your Healthcare Agent, you should discuss what types of treatments you would or would not want under different kinds of situations, for example:

- Whether or not you want life support initiated, continued, or removed if you are in a permanent coma

- Whether or not you want treatment initiated, continued, or eliminated if you are terminal

- Would you want artificial nutrition and hydration initiated, withheld, continued, or withdrawn, and under what considerations

Can My Healthcare Agent Overrule My Wishes Or Prior Treatment Instructions?

Your Healthcare Agent is obliged to make decisions based on your wishes. Suppose you clearly expressed particular wishes or gave particular treatment instructions. In that case, your Agent must follow those wishes or instructions unless they have a good faith basis for believing your wishes changed or do not apply to the situation.

Who Is Going To Pay Attention To My Agent?

All hospitals, nursing homes, doctors, and health care providers are legally required to provide your Healthcare Agent with the same information provided to you and honor the decisions by your Agent as if you made them. Suppose a hospital or nursing home objects to some treatment options (such as removing a particular therapy). They should tell you or your Agent **BEFORE or UPON ADMISSION.**

What Happens If My Healthcare Agent Is Not Available When Decisions Must Be Made?

You may appoint an **Alternate Healthcare Agent** to decide for you if your **Primary Healthcare Agent** is not accessible, unable, or unwilling to act when decisions must be made. Otherwise, the health care provider will decide for you to follow the instructions you gave when you were still able to. Any instructions you write on your **Healthcare Proxy (HCP)** will direct health care providers in such situations.

What Happens If I Change My Mind?

It is easy to rescind your Healthcare Proxy (HCP), change the person you have chosen as your Healthcare Agent, or change any instructions or limitations you have included on the HCP form. Just fill out a new HCP. Additionally, you can specify that your Healthcare Proxy expires on a specific date or if certain events happen. If not, your Healthcare Proxy will be effective for an indefinite period.

If your spouse was selected as your Healthcare Agent or Alternate Healthcare Agent and you are now divorced or legally separated, that appointment is automatically canceled. However, if you want your former spouse to remain your Agent, you may note this on your current HCP and date it or complete a new HCP identifying your former spouse.

Is My Healthcare Agent Legally Liable For Decisions Made On My Behalf?
No. Your Healthcare Agent is not liable for health care decisions made in good faith on your behalf. Also, they cannot be held responsible for your health care costs just because they are your Healthcare Agent.

Is a Healthcare Proxy The Same As a Living Will?
No, a **Living Will** provides particular instructions about health care decisions. You can put these instructions on your **Healthcare Proxy (HCP)** form. The HCP allows you to choose someone you trust to make health care decisions on your behalf. Contrary to a **Living Will, a Healthcare Proxy** does not require that you decide any decisions that may arise in advance. Instead, your Healthcare Agent may interpret your wishes as to medical circumstance changes and make decisions you could not have known that would have to be made.

Does A Healthcare Proxy Fit In With Advance Directives?
The term advance directive describes the documents you need should you become unable to carry out or make decisions on your behalf. Advance directives apply to both health care and financial decisions.

How Is a Healthcare Proxy Different From A Power Of Attorney?
A power of attorney (POA) is a document that permits you to designate an individual or organization to manage the property, financial, or medical affairs if you cannot. For instance, in a real estate transaction, you can give someone a temporary power of attorney to sign legal documents if you are not able to.

A general power of attorney gives the person or persons broad authority to make decisions. Those powers could include handling financial and business transactions, buying real estate or insurance, operating a business, or entering other legal agreements designated by the Grantor. However, all POAs are not equal. Each type gives your attorney-in-fact or the person who will be making decisions on your behalf varying levels of control. You may have a different person for financial power of attorney and another for Healthcare Proxy or Healthcare Power of Attorney.

Who Is Allowed To Override a Power of Attorney
The Grantor that created a power of attorney can cancel it, revoke or modify it so long as the Grantor has the mental capacity to do so. A court could cancel a power of attorney if it determined that the person appointed is abusing their ability and not acting in the person's (Grantor) best interests who created the Power of Attorney.

Power of Attorney vs. Living Will - the Healthcare Agent, appointed under a Healthcare Proxy, can make medical decisions, from giving consent to medical care to withdrawing treatment and medical interventions and allowing the patient to die naturally.

Where To Keep My Healthcare Proxy Form After It Is Signed?
Give the original to your attorney and a copy to your Healthcare Agent, doctor, and any family members or close friends you want. Always retain a copy in your wallet or purse with other important papers. Do not keep it in a location where no one can access it, such as a safe deposit box.
Note: bring a copy if you are to be admitted to the hospital, even for minor surgery, or if you undergo outpatient surgery.

Can I Use The Healthcare Proxy Form To Express My Wishes About Organ and Tissue Donation?
Complete the optional organ and tissue donation section on the Healthcare Proxy (HCP) form. Be sure to have the appropriate area witnessed by two people. You may specify that your organs and tissues be used for transplantation, research, or educational purposes. The proxy section should note any limitation(s) associated with your wishes.
Note: failure to include your wishes and instructions on your Healthcare Proxy (HCP) form will not mean you do not want to be an organ or tissue donor.

Can My Healthcare Agent Make Decisions About Organ and Tissue Donations?

Yes, your Healthcare Agent is permitted to make decisions after your death, but only those regarding organ and tissue donation. As noted on your **Healthcare Proxy (HCP)** form, your **Healthcare Agent** can make such decisions.

A Living Will

It is an expression of wishes for **End-of-Life Decision-making.** Many people have strong feelings about being artificially kept alive by machines, hydration, and feeding if there is no hope for recovery and death could be imminent. A **Living Will** should be a clear expression of your wishes and what you want to happen should those circumstances arise. You can create a Living Will while you are alive and well. *The Healthcare Agent appointed under your Healthcare Proxy (HCP) should follow your wishes for end-of-life decision-making if the situation arises and implement your wishes using the powers of the Healthcare Agent.*

APPENDIX A

We have included an exhaustive list of Must-Know Words and Phrases in this APPENDIX so that you and all parties can understand the terms and terminologies used by those administering **HEALTHCARE.**

"It's better to have it and not need it than to need it and not have it." - George Ellis

Must-Know Words and Phrases

Activities of Daily Living (ADL) - are basic tasks that people complete each day and are needed for basic functioning. It includes bathing, dressing, eating, toileting, and continence.

Acute Care - is a type of care provided to seniors for short-term medical conditions from which they are expected to recover. Upon full recovery, patients who need short-term care typically do not require daily attention to resume their everyday routines and lifestyle.

Adjuvant Therapy - additional treatment given to help lower the risk of cancer recurrence. Related conditions include chemotherapy, hormone therapy, and radiation.

Advance Directive - a legally binding document (if signed by witnesses or notarized) in which one makes one's health care goals, values, and preferences known. Different written advance directives are used in health care: the **Living Will, Healthcare Proxy, or MOLST/POLST.** Each fulfills a different role and, therefore, another need.

Alzheimer's Disease (AD) - is the most common kind of dementia. Alzheimer's Disease is a degenerative disease where the brain's function gradually declines and eventually causes death. The disease starts with short-term memory loss.

Ambulatory - refers to a person's capability for movement, i.e., Someone who is not confined to a bed or wheelchair.

Amyotrophic Lateral Sclerosis (ALS), also known as "Lou Gehrig's disease." - is a progressive disease in which the person's brain degenerates, causing muscle weakness and eventually death. Usually, the patient's cognitive functioning is unaffected.

Aging Life Care Manager/Geriatric Care Manager (GCM) - is a health care professional who has the ability and connections to assist seniors and their families in deciding on needed care, services providers of that care, and coordinating administration of that care.

Area Agency on Aging (AAA) - is a publicly funded agency that offers seniors programs and resources to assist in their care and ensure their rights are protected. The agency has local chapters located throughout the U.S.

Arthritis - is a joint disorder in which the joints become swollen and cause pain.

Assisted Living Facility (ALF) - provides a lower level of care than nursing homes. They generally allow the residents more freedom, requiring less skilled care and supervision than those in nursing homes. These facilities are also referred to as **"assisted living" (AL), "assisted living communities" (ALC), or "assisted living residences" (ALR).**

Asymptomatic - without any symptoms (or effects of a disease or illness).

Caregiver - a term used to describe an individual caring for, or helping to care for, a loved one.

Caregivers - provide non-medical care for seniors who need assistance with activities of daily living. Consideration may be provided in the home or a senior living community. Even though a caregiver is generally not a skilled medical professional, some may have specialized certifications or training.

Certified - Medicare and Medicaid outline requirements that a long-term care facility, home health agency, or hospice agency must satisfy. Medicare and Medicaid will only cover care costs if the facility is certified. Several long-term care insurance policies also have this same provision.

Certified Nursing Assistant (CNA) - a certified nursing assistant is a health care worker who works under the supervision of a nurse. They go through special training and generally work in nursing homes or hospitals. They offer patients non-medical support, such as help with eating, getting dressed, or cleaning their living space.

Chemo-brain - a **'mental cloudiness'** is a common side effect of chemotherapy.

Chemotherapy - is a treatment that uses oral or intravenous drugs to stop and kill rapidly growing cancer cells, also known as chemo.

Chronic - ongoing.

Chronic Obstructive Pulmonary Disease (COPD) - is a disease where the air pathways to the lungs restrict, limiting the ability to get air to the lungs. If the disease progresses, it could lead to death.

Code Status - refers to the level of medical intervention a patient wants to have if their heart or breathing stops. A code is called when the patient goes into cardiac or respiratory arrest. If the patient chooses **DNR,** that is also known as **NO CODE.** Numerous other codes vary based on the situation and health care setting, often with a name and a corresponding color code.

Combined "Living Will" and "Healthcare Proxy" documents - often referred to as **advance healthcare directives** combines the two documents into one document. Most documents used nowadays are of this type, including those encouraged by various state laws.

Companions - are people who provide in-home care and companionship for seniors. While companions do not offer medical care or hands-on care, they can perform household chores like cooking, cleaning, transportation, and errand-running. Individuals who need less assistance can hire companions for caregiving roles.

Complementary and alternative medicine (CAM) - treatments different from conventional medicine. Complementary treatment refers to practices or therapies used in conjunction with traditional approaches. Alternative methods refer to processes that are alternatives to conventional medicine. Examples can include special diets, acupuncture, and nutritional supplements.

Complete remission - refers to patients showing no signs of the disease.

Computerized Axial Tomography (CAT/CT) - A scan of the head or body that produces a cross-sectional image.

Congestive Heart Failure (CHF) - is the inability of the heart to provide sufficient blood for the body. It can lead to shortness of breath, swelling of the legs, and an inability to exercise. Contrary to some common opinions, it is not a heart attack.

Curative Care - unlike hospice, which focuses on symptom and pain management, curative care is any medical intervention seeking to treat patients to cure them, not just reduce their pain or stress. An example of curative care is chemotherapy, often used to cure cancer patients.

Dementia - is a symptom that refers to memory difficulties and other cognitive problems which interfere with everyday life. The deterioration of intellectual abilities includes a reduction in vocabulary, abstract thinking, judgment, memory, and physical coordination. Although there is no cure for dementia, there are treatments that can address some of the symptoms associated with dementia.

Discharge Planner - a discharge planner is a health care professional who delivers support to seniors and their families following the hospital or rehabilitation stay. They work with seniors to develop and coordinate a plan for post-recovery care.

A DNR (Do Not Resuscitate) or DNAR (Do Not Attempt Resuscitation) - is a medical order signifying that if the patient's heart stops beating (cardiac arrest), the medical staff should not initiate CPR (cardiopulmonary resuscitation) by chest compressions or electronic defibrillation but should allow death to occur naturally. Likewise, a DNR order means that if the patient stops breathing (respiratory arrest), the medical staff must not initiate artificial (mechanical) breathing by inserting a tube into the lungs (intubation) and then connecting that tube to a mechanical ventilator. Natural death is allowed to occur.

Durable Medical Equipment (DME) - is medical equipment used in a home to improve a senior's quality of life. Examples include wheelchairs, hospital beds, and catheters.

Edema - an accumulation of fluid in the tissues that leads to inflammation.

Electronic Health/Medical Record (EHR/EMR) - a system that maintains patients' health records. It makes it easier to transfer information across institutions and doctors' offices.

Emergency Medical Services (EMS) - generally means an ambulance with EMTs.

Emergency Medical Technician (EMT) - is a health care worker who responds to emergency medical situations. They are the workers that are staffing an ambulance. They have the training, but not as much as a nurse or doctor.

Exclusion - when an insurance company or a medical plan does not cover something, it is an exclusion. Health conditions, particular situations, equipment, services, or other costs may be considered exclusions.

Family Caregiver - a person that gives unpaid care to a family member. They help a relative who is ill, disabled, or dealing with a medical situation.

Geriatrician - a doctor, specializing in health care for elderly patients. These physicians treat seniors who have complex medical or social issues.

Health Insurance Portability and Accountability Act (HIPAA) - is a law that gives U.S. citizens certain privacy rights when it comes to health information. Specifically, HIPAA defines who can and cannot view personal health records and who has access to health information.

Healthcare Power of Attorney - you appoint someone to make healthcare decisions when you cannot do so for yourself.

Healthcare Proxy (HCP) - is a document in which an individual assigns another person or persons the authority to serve as their surrogate. Speaking on one's behalf when one cannot do so and representing the patient (principal or grantor) when medical decisions must be made.

Heart Disease - is a term that includes many diseases that affect the heart.

Home and Community-Based Services (HCBS) - services provided outside the institutionalized facility. This includes home health care and adult daycare.

Home Health Agency - a Medicare-certified organization that provides health care-related services in a person's home. They are accountable for coordinating and managing the care provided by home health aides to their clients. These agencies often provide nursing, social work, personal care, and various forms of therapy such as physical or occupational.

Home Health Aide (HHA) - provides primary care, typically for individuals in their own homes. This care can include waking, bathing, cleaning the living space, feeding, ensuring medications are taken, and assisting with any medical conditions. Most HHAs care for elderly clients.

Home Health Care (HCA) - is health care provided in the client's home. It might include home health aides, registered nurses, and skilled or unskilled care.

Hormone therapy - is a treatment that uses hormones to help slow or stop cancer growth. It is commonly used with breast and prostate cancer.

Hospice Care - is end-of-life care that focuses on making the patient as comfortable as possible while helping them cope with end-of-life problems. Specifically, hospice provides pain management, counseling, and comfort to patients and their family members. Hospice care lasts until the end of life. Depending on the recipient's wishes and circumstances, this can be provided in a facility, hospital, or private home.
Note: hospice care is for individuals who have a life-limiting diagnosis of six months or less, and it is covered under Medicare.

Hypertension - chronic high blood pressure can lead to other complications, such as a stroke.

Incontinence - the inability to control one's bladder.

Intensive Care Unit (ICU) - a part of the hospital for people in medically unstable conditions.

Licensed Practical Nurse (LPN) - a type of nurse who receives less training than a registered nurse and is more limited in the kind of care they can provide.

Life Plan Communities - a continuing care retirement community (CCRC) is a retirement community for the elderly that helps them live independently. As the elder's need for assistance increases, so does the level of care provided. Such communities usually have facilities that range from independent living apartments or condos to skilled nursing facilities. Seniors often move into continuing care retirement communities because they provide various levels of care in one place.

Life Support - refers to various medical technology/interventions utilized when one's vital organs, such as the brain, lungs, heart, or kidneys, are not functioning correctly. Life support serves as a bridge to help critically ill patients survive an acute experience until they recover.

Living Will - gives specific information about the procedures wanted, or not desired, to be performed if you become terminally ill. A Living Will is more specific in scope than a Healthcare Proxy (HCP) in that there are limited circumstances under which the Living Will takes effect. Your Healthcare Proxy cannot overrule decisions in your Living Will.

Long-Term Care (LTC) - is health care provided over an extended time for people who are chronically ill, disabled, or mentally disabled.

Long-Term Care Insurance (LCTI) - is an insurance plan separate from health insurance designed to cover the cost of long-term care. It typically needs to be purchased before the need for long-term care exists, as the plan's cost is based on the individual's age and health when purchasing the plan. Policy coverage will vary, so families need to understand components such as what type of care is covered, the amount of care covered, and if there are any elimination periods as part of the policy.

Long-Term Care Ombudsman - a person responsible for resolving issues between seniors, their families, and care facilities. Individuals living in nursing homes or long-term care facilities can file a complaint, and the independent, federally-funded Ombudsman Program will investigate the claim.

Macular Degeneration - is a condition that affects the ability to see, especially in the center of one's field of vision. This is a significant cause of sight loss in older adults.

Magnetic Resonance Imaging (MRI) - is a medical imaging device that uses radio and magnetic waves instead of radiation.

Medicaid - is a joint federal and state program managed by the state. It provides health insurance for those who are financially unable to cover their care costs. Although Medicaid covers a large percentage of the costs for those who live in nursing homes, it has specific federal requirements. Coverage and eligibility vary by state.

Medicare - is a federal program that provides health insurance coverage for seniors in the U.S that have paid into the benefit for a certain number of periods. Usually, individuals become eligible at 65, but individuals under 65 with specific disabilities may be qualified.

Medical/Physician's Order For Life-Sustaining Treatment - A Medical or Physician's Order For Life-Sustaining Treatment (MOLST/POLST) is a physician-initiated medical order beginning with a discussion between the patient and doctor centered on the patient's current condition. It assures that the patient's wishes regarding life-sustaining treatment will be carried out and is generally used for seriously ill patients. It is a durable form that travels with the patient and is honored across different care settings.

Myocardial Infarction (MI) - a heart attack.

Network - a group of doctors, hospitals, pharmacies, and other health care professionals that an individual has access to.

Nurse Practitioner (NP) - a licensed nurse that has completed graduate-level education and is allowed to conduct several of the functions that a doctor does, such as acting as a primary care provider and writing prescriptions.

Occupational Therapy (OT) - is a type of therapy that works with an individual to help them to perform the activities of daily living (ADLs) and instrumental activities of daily living (IADLs).

Organ donation - you can use a Healthcare Proxy (HCP) form to designate that your organs and tissues are used for transplantation, research, or educational purposes.

Out-of-Area Benefits - benefits offered outside the HMO's service area, usually only emergency services.

Out-of-Pocket Maximum - is the total amount of money a person must pay annually for their health insurance's deductibles and coinsurance. This cost is in addition to the insurance plan's premiums.

Out-of-Pocket Payments (OPP) - health care costs that are not covered by any insurance and have to be paid out of the insured's pocket.

Over the Counter (OTC) - is a term that refers to medication that does not require a prescription.

Palliative Care - is designed to reduce the physical and emotional pain that can come from having a severe illness. It is important to note that an individual does not need a terminal diagnosis for palliative care.

Patient Assessment - is an assessment of the patient usually conducted in health care facilities (e.g., assisted living facilities). They can determine the level of care that the patient requires.

Patient Days - are the number of days that a person is considered a patient in a health care facility. Specific insurance plans only include coverage for a certain number of patient days.

Personal Care Assistant (PCA) - is a person paid to provide those ill or chronically disabled assistance with their ADLs.

Personal Emergency Response System (PERS) - is an alarm system created to alert medical personnel of an emergency. It generally consists of a wireless transmitter that can be easily activated (pushing a button). These systems are typically portable and worn by or kept near the person who might need them.

Physician Assistant (PA) - is a healthcare professional licensed to work under a physician's supervision. The PA can conduct physical exams, write prescriptions, and diagnose and treat illnesses, among other functions.

Plan of Care - a written plan of medical services and care a person needs, typically prepared by the individual's doctor.

Power of Attorney (POA) or Durable Power of Attorney (DPA) - authorizes the designated person to make financial decisions. However, this person cannot use the POA or DPA to make health care decisions. You must complete a Healthcare Proxy (HCP) for that purpose. In certain states, the phrase **'Healthcare Power of Attorney'** will clarify that the term is for the express purpose of health care decisions.

Preferred Provider Organization (PPO) - is a managed-care organization contracting with health care providers to provide discounted rates to patients covered by its insurance plan.

Primary Care Physician/Provider (PCP) - is a health care provider that provides care to a person in an outpatient setting, both preventative and curative (e.g., regular check-ups and advice on fundamental medical issues).

Private Pay - refers to people paying for care out of pocket instead of through public or private insurance plans.

Registered Nurse (RN) - a licensed health care professional who provides care in various environments. The RN can conduct tests and other medical procedures under a physician's supervision, but they cannot prescribe medications.

Rider - an add-on provision to an insurance policy that details additional benefits the policyholder will receive for an additional cost.

Skilled Nursing Facility (SNF) - a facility that provides a high level of nursing care. It is also known as a nursing home.

Social Security Disability Insurance (SSD/SSDI) - is a federal insurance program that covers people who cannot work due to a disability. The aid is given in a monthly stipend and is not dependent on income.

Supplemental Security Income (SSI) - is a federal program that provides stipends to low-income and above 65, blind, or otherwise disabled.

Terminal/Life-Limiting Illness - there is no standard clinical definition for the terminally ill. However, the word is often loosely used to refer to a patient's prognosis with an incurable fatal disease in contemporary medicine. In **hospice care,** it is often identified as an illness expected to leave the afflicted six months or less to live. Clinicians suggest that **terminal illness** be applied only to the condition of patients who experienced clinicians expect to die from a lethal, progressive disease despite appropriate treatment and in a relatively short time, usually measured in days, weeks, or at most several months.

The Centers for Medicare and Medicaid Services (CMS) - the federal agency that controls Medicare and Medicaid programs. It is also in charge of CMS regulations and certifications.

Veteran's Affairs (VA) - a government veteran benefits program. Health care insurance is a benefit option and some additional benefits that can help cover the cost of long-term care.

Visiting Nurses - are registered nurses who give in-home care. They provide medical, rehabilitative, and hospice care.

APPENDIX B

Life-Sustaining Treatments

If you have any questions about life-sustaining treatment, speak to a medical professional, preferably one on the patient's health care team. Like any procedure, one must compare the benefits to the risks.

Cardiopulmonary Resuscitation (CPR)

Such medical procedures are used when a person's heart or breathing stops. CPR is used to restart a heart and restore breathing. It can often save lives when performed on an otherwise healthy person after an accident or heart attack. The success rate is much lower when used on individuals with a terminal disease. Common procedures during CPR are:

- Chest compression

- Electric shock

- Injecting medication into the heart or open chest

- Inserting a tube to open the airway

- Mouth-to-mouth resuscitation

Mechanical Ventilator

It is a machine used to help people breathe when they cannot live effectively on their own. Patients will be placed on a ventilator (sometimes called a respirator), which puts air in their lungs. Tubing is inserted into the mouth and sent down the windpipe. Mechanical ventilation is frequently used for a few days to a few weeks to help individuals breathe. To be placed on a ventilator can help people with acute or chronic, stable conditions.

Mechanical ventilation improves oxygen supply when a person is dying but does not improve their condition. It may prolong life until another body system fails, and the overall quality of the person's life is not enhanced.

Artificial Nutrition and Hydration

This replaces ordinary food and liquid intake when a patient can no longer swallow. A line is placed directly into the nose, stomach, upper intestine, or vein. Artificial nutrition and hydration could save lives when used until the body can heal itself. Unfortunately, it cannot reverse the course of a disease.

The Organ Donor

Becoming an organ donor is a selfless act. It is a form of generosity that continues even when you no longer are here. Organ donors have the opportunity to give others a new lease on life. Frequently when recipients have run out of other options. If you decide to become an organ donor, you may unknowingly become the hero of someone you have never met.

When Should You Decide To Become An Organ Donor?
In life, some of the most important decisions to make are sometimes the ones you struggle with the most. This can be true when you decide if you should sign up to become an organ donor. Even though it can be challenging, making this decision is so important. It lands with all the other choices you should be making about your healthcare decisions.

What is Needed to Be an Organ Donor?
If you are considering being an organ donor, remember that certain requirements need to be met. Meeting the following requirements will ensure that you have done everything you need to become a donor after you pass away.

- You are over the age of 18

- You do not have active cancer

- You do not have a systemic infection

Note: if you are under the age of 18 and wish to be a donor, you might still be able to do so, depending on your state law. But, your family will have to give their blessing.

Pros and Cons of Becoming an Organ Donor
Whenever you have a difficult decision in life, assessing the pros and cons may help you feel better about whatever decision you ultimately come to.

PROS - there are many positive aspects to being an organ donor.

- The ability to save a life, or several lives

- Comfort for your family. Once someone has passed away, most families report feeling an incredible feeling of peace, knowing that their loved one contributed to the well-being of others.

- You do not need to be an exact match. Blood and tissue types are typically more important than the preconceived notion that you must be a perfect match.

- Ability to advance research. If you contribute your body to science for medical research, especially if you have a rare disease. It may allow for treatments or cures to be developed.

- Help in training the future medical community. Your donation means students can practice their techniques and conduct research to enhance their skills and know-how.

CONS - of course, there are drawbacks to every decision made.

- Donors will be kept on life support. Without organs, donors may be kept on life-support, which is painful for family members.

Note: Losing a loved one is difficult, and the thought of the organs being donated can be a callous process for some people to come to terms with.

Autopsies

An autopsy is a thorough dissection of a deceased person to determine why they died. In coping with the sudden loss of a loved one, you may find comfort in getting answers to the WHY at this challenging time. But, you should also know that autopsies do not always have to be done. It is usually both a medical and a legal process if you need one. Laws differ state by state.

You can request an autopsy if you have questions about how a family member died. Sometimes doctors will ask permission to do one if they have questions.

Coroners and Medical Examiners
Each local government has an official who records deaths. They are called the coroner or medical examiner. Most states require medical examiners to be doctors. Coroners may be doctors, but they do not have to be. Coroners are usually elected officials, and many do not have medical training. So, when an autopsy is required, they rely on a medical examiner.

What Happens In an Autopsy?
A physician examines the remains. They remove internal organs for testing and collect samples of tissue and bodily fluids such as blood. The examination usually takes 1 to 2 hours. Often, these experts can figure out the cause of death at that time. Some situations might require you to wait until the laboratory can complete additional tests to look for signs of drugs, poisons, or disease, which can take several days or weeks.

Once completed, the doctor will report an exact cause of death and how they think it happened, whether someone died from natural causes, accidents, etcetera.

When Is an Autopsy Necessary?
Though laws vary, nearly all states call for an autopsy when someone dies suspiciously, unusual, or unnatural. Many states require one when a person dies without a doctor present. Additionally, some states require an autopsy if the cause of death is suspected of being a public health threat.

When Is It Optional?

A doctor might ask to allow an autopsy if a loved one died of an unexpected illness. They are usually trying to learn more about what happened, either to ease your mind, learn if other family members might be in danger of the same thing, or find out something that might help other patients. In some cases, a person's condition in life can only be diagnosed after they die. For instance, doctors can learn that someone has Alzheimer's disease only after examining the brain at an autopsy. It is for the family to decide whether to allow it.

Note: some private firms do autopsies for a fee in addition to public officials.

Family Wishes and Faith

Some faith traditions discourage autopsies, believing a person's body should be kept whole or otherwise left alone after death. Or they may say burial should not be delayed.

Several states have laws that honor religious objections. Medical examiners sometimes change how they perform an autopsy out of respect for the family's beliefs. But states still require one when it is needed to investigate a crime or head off a threat to public health. Most examinations should not delay a funeral or prevent viewing of the body during a service. Funeral directors can usually hide any signs of the autopsy with clothing.

What Does Disposition Of Last Remains Mean?

Most people plan for significant events in their lives. For weddings, much attention is given to the location, day, time, flowers, cake, photographer, wedding favors, seating chart, etcetera. These decisions are not typically made quickly. It is not uncommon for events like these to take a year or more to plan properly. Aside from wanting the event to succeed, people wish their personalities reflected in every detail.

The funeral service, memorial service, or celebration of life is the last significant event in a person's life. That is when family and friends gather to say goodbye, remember good times, and reflect on the legacy the person left behind. If you want to ensure that your last big event occurs precisely as you envisioned, you might draw up a **Statement of Disposition of Remains (SDR).**

Specify Your End-of-Life Details
A Statement of Disposition of Remains (SDR) can contain information about:

- The method you want your physical body to be handled after passing away. You can specify if you will be buried (including the exact location and the type of casket), cremated (including what is to be done with your ashes), or entombed. People have been buried with material possessions and had their ashes shot off in firework displays!

- If any, what type of ceremony do you want to celebrate your life (including no event at all). If you want a formal funeral with a wake, specify which funeral home you prefer. Perhaps you want a more casual event such as a memorial service or celebration of life where attendees are encouraged to wear tie dye clothing and share their memories during the ceremony. You can choose to have a very public event or a private event with close family members.

- Organ or tissue donation information. This document can provide general direction for your loved ones to follow or contain specific details about how you want everything handled. Be clear, so your loved ones will have less to agree on. It is the last chance you have to leave your mark, reminding your loved ones of the type of person you were.

Understanding Disposition Options

The word disposition refers to how a person's remains are managed. Standard methods of disposition are listed below. A funeral director can answer questions to help you make a choice that is right for you.

- **Earth Burial** - this refers to an inground placement of your remains. It is generally in a casket, although some cemeteries allow the remains to be buried without coffins, often to meet the requirements of a specific religious or cultural group. This form of internment may or may not involve embalming the deceased's body. Earth burial requires a cemetery plot and has fees for opening and closing the grave and perpetual graveside care.

- **Above-Ground Burial (Entombment**) - requires purchasing a crypt within a mausoleum specifically designed for entombment. A funeral director can advise on the availability and options in your community.

- **Cremation** - remains are reduced to a powder-like substance through intense heat from a furnace known as a cremation chamber or retort. The refined substance (remains) is placed in a temporary container. Before the remains are returned to the family, they usually are transferred to an urn for permanent containment.

- **Not Always Without Ceremony** - many people believe that only two basic choices exist at the time of death: immediate cremation of the body or a complete funeral, including viewing, followed by burial. However, there are several options available to those who prefer cremation.

  Cremation and burial are methods of caring for the body and are just one part of a funeral. Like burial, cremation may occur after the funeral where the casket is present at a place of worship or funeral chapel.

- **Alkaline Hydrolysis** - a relatively new method of disposition (not available in every state). This process involves using pressure, heat, and lye to break the remains down into their chemical components, resulting in a liquid and ash which can be returned to loved ones. Advocates of this process say it is a more ecologically friendly option than cremation.

AFTERWORD

Thank you for reading,

**Proxy Information For You And
Your Healthcare Agent**

We hope you enjoyed this
Life Knowledge Media USA Publication

Thank you again, valued reader,
and we hope to meet you again on another book.

ABOUT THE AUTHOR

Pierre Mouchette is the Founder and CEO of Real Property Experts LLC. He is a graduate of New York University, with a Master's in Business Administration, a Certificate in Real Estate Law - Fairfield University - CT, a Graduate of the Realtors Institute - CT, and held licensing as a Real Estate Broker, and a Mortgage Broker.

Pierre is currently authoring Books, Booklets, How-to-Articles, and Guides in retirement. Pierre has an extensive background in real estate investment, business management, and sales, supplemented by decades of hands-on experience in building systems engineering, development, evaluation, and various analytical engineering studies.

Pierre launched Real Property Experts in 2013 to simplify real estate investing by connecting investors through innovative technology using background knowledge and experience. In 2018, Pierre created THE SYNCHRONICITY INVESTOR, a real estate website to facilitate world-class solutions for real estate investors and investment businesses.

During the winter of 2021, Pierre created Enviro | Life Publications to bring Environmental and LIfe Knowledge to a growing TSI audience. Exploring the Internet and using all sources available, this entity will bring to our audience, through its Research, Information that is Transparent and easy to understand, thereby making them more Knowledgeable.

<table>
<tr><td colspan="2" align="center">Life Knowledge Media USA

- presents -

An Enviro | Life Knowledge Publication</td></tr>
<tr><td colspan="2">MISCELLANEOUS</td></tr>
<tr><td></td><td>SBA Disaster Loans</td></tr>
<tr><td></td><td>The Ultimate Guide To An Enlightened End</td></tr>
<tr><td></td><td>THE LEGACY - A Guide For Family Continuation</td></tr>
<tr><td></td><td>Proxy Information For You And Your Healthcare Agent</td></tr>
</table>